Pitching Yourself For PA School

The Physician Assistant School Application Essay

"Your personal statement tells the story *of* you, not just a story *about* you."

Dr. Oren Berkowitz

The stories and essays contained in this book are original works of fiction. Any resemblance to real persons, alive or dead, or to previously written essays is purely coincidental

DEDICATION

To my dear family, including those yet to come into
our lives.
And to my students, who continuously inspire me
and make me proud.

Also by Oren Berkowitz

The Brain Surgeon
A medical fiction novel

www.DrOrenBerkowitz.com

CONTENTS

PREFACE

How to Use This Book

SELLING YOURSELF WELL AND PITCHING YOUR application is a challenge that could mean the difference between getting an interview and having your application put aside. This book is a manual for physician assistant (PA) school applicants. The personal statement is a longstanding tradition of school applications and it is the chance to tell your story and fill in the blanks that the rest of your application leaves open. This manual is meant to help you better understand how to tell your story for the complex and competitive process of PA school application and acceptance. The advice is delivered through the fictional story of a retired professor and a PA school applicant. The characters are fictional. The essays discussed are also works of fiction and only meant to serve as examples of common essays and how an applicant might be perceived by the admissions committee. The author has woven a blend of anecdotal and evidence based advice into the fictional story and reference sources are listed at the end of the book.

This book is not a how-to manual or a style guide. There is no cookie cutter template to follow that will get you into PA school. The cognitive elements of the application (GPA, GRE, etc.) remain the most important factors for getting screened in. The personal essay is part of the non-cognitive factors that help programs round out their decisions about who might be a good fit for them and for the PA profession. When someone reads your essay, they want to get a sense of your personality, motivation, and fit. Since programs want a variety of student types, every essay has the potential to shine a light on who you are. The story in this book is meant to help you get to know a fictional applicant named Sarah, and then see how Sarah learns to translate her personality, motivation, and fit into a finalized essay, even while using many of the common PA school essay themes, which are discussed in the story.

The author is a founding faculty member of a PA program but does not endorse any particular PA program in this manual and strongly advises the reader to perform personal due diligence whenever applying to a PA program. This manual is a guidebook and does not constitute a guarantee or a promise of acceptance into any PA program.

"Writing is easy. All you have to do is cross out the wrong words."

Mark Twain

INTRODUCTIONS

SARAH THREW HER ARM IN BETWEEN THE BUS doors just as they were closing. She climbed in and shrugged her shoulders at the puzzled bus driver. She probably could have just knocked on the bus door without putting her arm at risk of serious injury but she was nervous and didn't want to be late to her meeting with Professor Rosen.

They had agreed to meet a few blocks away, at one of the campus coffee houses. She wasn't exactly sure how to greet him. Is 'Professor' the most appropriate, she thought? Or doctor? Or did he revert to some casual, grandfatherly, first name basis after he retired? She decided to go with 'Professor'.

Sarah was lucky to get this meeting. Sarah worked part-time at a rehab facility and she would sometimes stick around and play the piano in the recreation room, giving her a chance to chat with people. A family member of one of her patients started up a conversation with her one day, asking about her interests and plans. When Sarah told her that her goal was to become a PA, she mentioned that her cousin is a professor who recently retired, who had run a PA program at a nearby university for many years. She contacted him about meeting with her and he agreed to it.

Sarah swung open the doors to the coffee shop and immediately recognized Professor Rosen from his pictures online. She quickly checked the time on her cell phone to make sure she wasn't late. She had arrived five minutes early but he was already there. She walked over to his table slowly, waiting for him to notice her. He glanced up from his cappuccino and gave her a big smile as he stood up from his chair and waived her over. Sarah shook his hand.

"Nice to meet you, Professor Rosen," she said. "Thank you so much for taking the time to meet with me."

"Absolutely no problem, Sarah," he answered. "It is a pleasure to help someone interested in joining the ranks of our profession. And besides, it is nice to still be able to share some wisdom now that I have left the classroom."

Professor Rosen had a medium length salt and pepper beard. He had a canopy of bushy eyebrows over brown eyes. The thin hair on his head matched his beard and he wore a dark blazer with dark jeans.

"I can start by telling you a little bit about myself and then we can jump into how I might be able to advise you. Does that sound good?" He asked.

"Yes, perfect," she answered.

"Okay. So, I was the program director of a PA program for many years. I started my career as a clinical PA in the emergency room, back in the age of the dinosaurs. I used to be a medic in the army and I got my PA certificate after I left the service. Back then they mostly gave out certificates and I had to get my bachelor's degree on my own."

"Oh, really?" she interrupted.

"Yup. It is actually a fairly new decision on behalf of the profession to make the entry level degree a master's degree. Keep in mind the profession has been around since 1967, so it is both well-developed and still evolving."

Professor Rosen took a sip of his cappuccino to regain his train of thought.

"So several years into my clinical work," he continued, "I discovered a passion for teaching and I decided to go back to school and get a doctorate in education. After that, I transitioned into my first faculty position in a PA program and had my hand in every role over several years until I became the program director. I have advised over a thousand students over the decades and gone through thousands more applications. I just retired a couple of years ago. So that is a little bit of my story, why don't you tell me a little bit about yourself? What are your dreams, your aspirations? Let's figure out how I can help you."

I felt intimidated. A nervous smile and chuckle came over me. I didn't know where to start. He must have sensed my hesitation.

"Okay, how about this," he said. "Let's start with your academic career. What year are you in and what is your major?"

"I am a senior," she answered, "I am majoring in biology."

"Was it always biology?" he asked.

"Yes," she said. "I have known that I wanted to be a PA for a long time, now. I actually joined the pre-PA club at school."

"Great," he said, "So tell me more about why are you interested in becoming a PA?"

"I had a chance to shadow a couple of the PAs through the pre-health professions office at school. They took me to their primary care clinic and I fell in love with what they were doing. It was the first time I had ever seen a Patient-Centered Medical Home. They seemed to spend more time talking to patients and educating them than any physician I shadowed. Especially, Pat. She became a role model for me. She was everybody's go-to person in the clinic and seemed really dedicated to involving all of the team members in her patient care plans."

"That's good," he said, "I am glad to hear that someone took you under her wing and showed you what PAs are all about. Is there anything else about the PA profession in particular that you like?"

"I also love the fact that I can change specialties and work in different settings over the course of my career," she said. "It really seems like a great way to care for many different populations and for me to continue learning and growing."

"Good," Professor Rosen nodded, "You seem to have the right idea about PAs, overall. Did you know that a typical PA switches specialties about three times during their career?"

"No, I didn't know that, but that sounds very appealing. As a PA, you have the chance to try so many different things"

"That's right. I know one PA who started her career in obstetrics and gynecology and then switched to dermatology, and is now a liver specialist! There are lots of opportunities." Professor Rosen said as he leaned back in his chair.

"Alright," he continued, "so are you mainly getting your clinical hours at the rehab facility?"

"Yes. I work there as a nurse's aide, part time."

"That's good. And what do you for fun?"

"Fun?" Sarah asked. She raised her eyebrows and looked off to the corner of the room as she thought about the question. "I don't know, I don't really have much time outside of school and work."

"I understand," he said, nodding his head as if he expected me to say that. "But what would you be doing if you did have time? Everyone has interests outside of their daily routine."

"Well, I like to play the piano. I had a group of friends that I would play with but I haven't done it in a while. Now I practice after work at the rehab facility by playing for the residents."

"Oh, that's very nice. Anything else? What occupies you during your summer breaks?"

"I still go to summer camp!" I laughed. "Actually, I work now at the summer camp I went to as a kid. I got my EMT certificate and I work in the camp's health clinic. It's a lot of fun."

"That does sound like fun," he said with a smile. "Have you started putting your application together on the central application service?"

"Yes, I have," she said while nodding, "It is a little intimidating, there are so many pieces to it."

"That's true," he said, "Do you have any questions about the application process so far?"

Sarah adjusted the glasses on her face.

"I guess," she started, "my first question would be, which part of the application is the most important to PA programs?"

He smiled and raised his cappuccino in the air.

"That is the million dollar question, isn't it," he said, "but the funny thing is, the answer is no mystery…"

"The personal statement," she confirmed, while nodding her head.

"NO!" he snapped with a smirk on his face while wagging his finger at her. Sarah dropped the spiral binder she had been taking notes in onto the table and stared at him, not sure what to say.

"Too many prep books, blogs, and consultants have misled you to think that you can write your way into PA school," he continued, "but nothing could be further from the truth. The most well studied and proven aspect of your application, that predicts success in PA school and on the boards, are your grades! Your grade point average, GRE, coursework, etc.; we call these cognitive measures. Like the old dictum says, 'past performance predicts future performance.'"

"But isn't the essay how you get to know me, as a person? Shouldn't that be the most important part of the application?" Sarah asked.

"Sure, the personal essay is important," he said, "but you can't write your way out of poor performance."

"Grades aren't the only things that matter," she said, incredulously, "personal experience, empathy, passion… all those things should matter more."

"You are absolutely right," he said reassuringly, "those things are weighed, and heavily. But the bottom line is, if someone can't pass the PA coursework, they won't become a PA. Only once someone has proven, on paper, that they have what it takes to pass the curriculum, will they be given a further look to find out about experience, empathy, and passion. Those are called non-cognitive measures. It all comes together as part of the holistic process."

"So then what's the point?" she shrugged,

"why write an essay at all? PA programs should just accept people based on their grades."

"Don't take it the wrong way," he laughed, "the personal statement is very important and it counts for a lot. Most of the PA school applicants have wonderful grades and the personal statement is what can set them apart from each other. And research has shown that the majority of PA schools think that the personal essay is valuable and is primarily used to determine who to invite for an interview. If an applicant doesn't demonstrate their experience, empathy, and passion, they are not very likely to get an interview. But if they do this well, and have good grades, their chances go way up."

"Well, how do I know if my grades are good enough?" she asked.

"That is another great question," he answered, "and keep in mind that different PA programs have different criteria for what they consider to be adequate grades. Some programs will even advertise minimum standards or the typical grade point average, also known as GPA, of their applicants on their website. So you want to make sure that you aren't too far off from those. In the meantime, let's take a look at what the average accepted PA school applicant looks like on paper. Here are some numbers based on recent reports from CASPA."

Professor Rosen clicked on his laptop and spun the screen around for Sarah to see. She pushed her glasses up on her nose and started going through the numbers row by row...

Characteristics of Students Who Recently Matriculated Into PA School[1]

Female	70%
Male	30%
Median Age	25
White	75%
Hispanic	7%
Asian	8%
Black	3%
Other or mixed	7%
Most common major	Biology
#healthcare hours	4-5,000
Science GPA	3.46
Overall GPA	3.52
GRE percentile scores	
Verbal	68%
Quantitative	62%
Analytical	61%

[1] Adapted from aggregate data reports (2012-2014) available at: CASPA Resources for Programs. http://paeaonline.org/caspa/program-resources/. Accessed December 26, 2016.

"These look like impressive numbers," she said, while emitting a sigh.

"They are very impressive," he agreed, "and they are getting more competitive with every year that passes. Lately, there have been a little over 21,000 applications per year with just over 7,000 students matriculating, which comes to a competition of around three applicants for every seat, depending on the year. This rate fluctuates slightly but it has been trending upwards over the past decade. Also, keep in mind, that the competition is vastly different between programs. Some of the legacy programs and also those in highly desirable schools and locations can have 10-30 applicants per seat. So you understand, even if you are a competitive applicant with a brilliant personal statement, it is very important to apply to more than one program and to spread your applications over several different levels of competitiveness."

"Like have some safety schools?" she asked.

"Exactly," he said.

"So, about the grades," she asked nervously, "can you tell me a little bit more about making the cut?"

"Sure," he said, sensing that there was more to Sarah's question, "and before I forget, I am going to grab another coffee. Do you want something? It looks like you didn't get anything before sitting down."

"Oh, that's right," she said, realizing that she forgot to get a drink. "I'll have a regular coffee, please. Thank you."

Professor Rosen got in line to order the drinks while Sarah scribbled away furiously at her notepad. She didn't notice her phone vibrating or how late she was for her evening study group. Professor Rosen came back to the table with two coffees and a giant blueberry muffin that he promptly cut in two pieces and shared with Sarah. He launched right into his explanation.

"There are several ways for an admissions committee to look at an applicant's transcript," he started, as he picked up his half of the muffin. He gestured for Sarah to take a piece of the muffin as well. "The GPA is reported in several ways, including: an overall number, a science average, and subject matter averages. The overall GPA on its own doesn't tell you enough about performance because, for example, someone might not have consistently good grades but they average out well, or they may not be taking challenging courses. How do you like the muffin?"

Sarah raised her eyebrows and nodded her head, "Uh, it's good, yeah, thank you."

He stared at her for a moment to see if she would tell him what was really on her mind about her grades, but she didn't take the bait.

He continued, "Let's say a student struggled in their first year; the transcript better show improvement over time. We would be more forgiving of an applicant who got a few C grades in their freshman year but then improved in subsequent years than we would be of someone who seems to always get several C grades at every level. Remember that undergraduate coursework generally starts with easier, introductory courses in the first couple of years and becomes progressively more difficult in the later years, so if a student's performance isn't consistent or improving with time, it makes us think that they cannot handle high level coursework. Also, don't forget that we usually weigh the science grades more heavily than the other grades, so most programs have a minimum science GPA requirement, usually around 3.0. But don't rely on the bare minimum, because you see from the stats that most students who end up getting accepted into a PA program have a higher GPA than that minimum."

Sarah squirmed around in her chair. She began tapping her pen on her notebook. Professor Rosen just went ahead and asked her.

"So, tell me about your grades," he probed.

"Um, I mean, they're not bad," she said, "I am definitely above the minimum science GPA of 3.0 and I am pretty close to that overall average GPA you showed me. But I did have some trouble in my freshman year. I see what you mean about some admissions committees being forgiving of that, but I really want to get into a good PA program and I don't want it to ruin my chances, especially given how competitive it is."

"I get it," he said, "so what happened?"

"Well, like you said," she started, "I was having some trouble adapting to my new college life. I thought I could approach class like I did in high school but when I started my first science course with three hundred other students, I couldn't keep up. I was also trying to develop a social life at the same time and I was frequently traveling home to help out my grandmother, who has Parkinson's disease. I got a few C grades that first year before I was able to get a handle on things. But my grades did get a lot better my sophomore year."

"Well, I might be able to help you there," he said, "it is a common story that many students experience and that's where your personal statement comes into play. That's your chance to tell your story and explain yourself on paper. You don't want to make the common mistake that so many students make when they write their essay and don't talk about the challenges they have overcome. For example, if someone's application shows any academic discipline, extended leave of absence, or undergraduate credits taken at many different institutions, it will raise flags. These things are easily noticed by an admissions reader and if they are not addressed in the essay, the reader might think the applicant is unpredictable or hiding something. Have you started writing your statement?"

"Yes, I have," she said, "I began a rough

draft but it is not finished yet. I didn't mention anything about my freshman year, so far."

"Have you asked anyone to look at it yet?" He asked.

"No," she replied, "I haven't really thought about that, yet."

"Why don't you email it to me and we can talk about it more next week," he suggested, "It is so important to have other people read your essay. No matter how well you write, you can never fully predict how you will appear to someone else on paper. I always recommend having two people read your essay: one who knows you well and one who barely knows you at all. Both of them should give you style and grammar edits but the one who knows you well can help you sell yourself by pointing out your accomplishments and helping you tell your story. The one who hardly knows you at all can give you honest and open feedback on how you appear on paper and whether your essay brings out your personality, motivations, and fit. So, anyway, I look forward to reading it and we can meet again for coffee next week."

"That sounds great!" she said, "Thank you so much for all of your help. See you then."

THE ROUGH DRAFT

"OK, SARAH," HE STARTED AS SHE SAT DOWN AT the table next to him. He had indicated for her to sit beside him in order for them to look at his laptop computer screen together. Today he had two coffees and a blueberry muffin ready for them when Sarah arrived.

"I reviewed the rough draft of your essay," he continued, "I understand that you are not finished yet, but let's take a look at what you've got, together. Just to reiterate, the application instructions from central application website are as follows:"

"In the space provided write a brief statement expressing your motivation or desire to become a physician assistant. Keep your statement general as the same essay will be sent to all schools you will apply to. **Even if you only plan to apply to one program, do NOT make your essays school specific as you may decide to apply to additional programs at a later date, and once you submit your application your essay can NOT be edited or changed. Maximum Length: 5,000 Characters"** [2]

"Now let's review what you have so far of your essay:"

---

[2] CASPA Essay Requirements.
https://portal.caspaonline.org/caspaHelpPages/frequently-asked-questions/additional-information/narrative-personal-statement-information/index.html. Accessed December 26, 2016.

Sarah's essay. Rough draft

My shift at the rehab facility had started just like any other, but I could never have imagined what would happen next. Mrs. S, who I had taken care of for a few weeks already, finished her dinner and asked me to turn on her favorite TV show. Just as she was settling in to her bed and I had turned around to leave the room, I heard a loud crash. I rushed back to her and she was struggling to breath. The crash I heard was the sound of her bedside alarm clock hitting the ground as she flailed her arms around frantically. I hit the code button on the wall to summon help. Her face was turning blue and she quickly lost consciousness. I remembered my CPR training and immediately launched into emergency mode. I couldn't detect any breathing and if she had a pulse, it was too faint to discern. I jumped onto the bed with her and started doing chest compressions. My colleagues had rushed into the room by now and were opening up a crash cart. Just as I was about twenty or thirty chest compressions in, I heard a mild popping sound and Mrs. S suddenly began to cough. I stopped doing compressions and Mrs. S coughed up a big grape that must have come from her fruit cup! She started breathing normally again and the ambulance arrived and took her to the hospital, just to get checked out, but she turned out to be just fine.

I always knew that I wanted to work in the medical field. Like most people, I wasn't always sure how I would respond in the face of a true emergency. Would I freeze up, or would I rise to the occasion? After that moment with Mrs. S, I knew that I would be able to handle myself in a medical emergency and it truly solidified my longstanding desire to become a PA.

I knew that I wanted to become a PA as soon as I got a chance to shadow one in her primary care clinic. I saw how compassionate she was and how much time she would take talking to her patients and educating them. I knew that I wanted a job where I would be able to give that extra level of care and attention. I love the idea of working as part of a team and I think that the PA profession would give me the right balance of autonomy while still having people to go to if it is ever needed. I am a team player and I really think that PA is the right fit for me.

The entire time he was reading over her essay, Sarah kept her eyes on the ground. She had that feeling of severe angst that comes over you when someone else is looking at your work, especially when they have a critical eye. Professor Rosen was a master teacher, though, and rather than tell Sarah whether he thought her essay was *good* or *bad*, he opted for a different pedagogy.

"Now," he said after a short pause, "I am going to pull up two different essays from former students. These are short essays that we asked our students to write in preparation for a global health rotation. You see, at our program, we offered a clinical elective in global health. During their clinical rotations, we would send two to three students at a time for nearly a month to very remote and medically underserved areas. These were usually Central American countries where only Spanish was spoken and students travelled with medical NGOs; do you know what an NGO is?"

"Um, I've heard of it but I am not sure what it stands for."

"Non-Government Organization. Basically a humanitarian group that does not answer to any specific government or health system. Anyway, the students would travel with these NGO groups in conditions that were often difficult. No air conditioning, limited electricity, sometimes no toilet plumbing, and forget about any internet or wireless connections, for days on end. And of course there was the risk of contracting an illness like diarrhea, malaria, dengue fever, etc. These were not tropical beach paradise vacations. Sometimes, you could really wonder what on earth would drive a student to do this, but it was a physical and emotional challenge that was incredibly rewarding and created lessons learned for life. These rotations were tremendously popular. But we needed to think very hard about who we would send on theses rotations, given the liabilities and risks associated."

"So you made it into, like, a competition? The best essays would go?" Sarah asked, squinting her eyes a bit.

"So, actually," he continued, while waiving his hand in front of the computer, as if attempting to manually redirect her thoughts, "we wanted to send as many students as we could, without necessarily ranking them. So it wasn't so much a competition, but it was very important that the student could make it clear to us what their motivations were and what they expected to get from the rotation. It was more of a filtering process. To use an extreme example, we wanted to make sure that the student didn't expect to be spending a month in a Central American all-inclusive resort, working on their tan at the hotel, in between seeing patients in an air conditioned clinic."

"Yeah, but that just sounds silly," Sarah interjected, "people probably know what they are signing up for? I mean, of course they won't think that they are just going for a vacation."

"Well," he laughed, "you are probably right for most of the students. But you would be surprised at how many essays we received from students about wanting to go and visit relatives who live in the same country, or asking if they can bring their girlfriend along on the trip. That is not what this was about. But like I said, those were the more extreme cases and they got filtered out pretty rapidly. We were mostly trying to find the more nuanced themes in those essays. If we really needed to rank students because we just didn't have enough slots available, it would be more about their academic standing and their clinical schedule than the essay. For example, if a student was struggling in cardiology, we might recommend that they spend their elective in a cardiology specialty rotation to improve their competencies, rather than do a global health rotation."

"Ok, I think I understand what you are getting at, the essay won't make up for poor performance," she said.

"Exactly right," he said, pointing his finger in the air.

"And it will weed out the ridiculously bad ones," she said.

"Right," he laughed.

"So then, what exactly are you looking for in an essay? I still don't understand why you don't just pick people based on their grades? If everybody is writing with the same goal in mind, how are you really able to tell all of those essays apart?" she asked while shaking her head in frustration.

Professor Rosen put his hand up and counted off on three fingers.

"Personality, motivation, and fit," he said,

let's get right into it, here are two examples. They are very different from each other. We will talk about why that is and what you think about them after we read through:"

Kelsey's global health rotation essay

Rosa was 93 years old. I visited her every other weekend while I was volunteering at the Sunny Horizons nursing home. We would play Rummy and sometimes I would read to her. But what she loved to do most of all was tell me stories about her childhood in Honduras. She grew up in a remote mountain village near the town of Olanchito. Her family had cows and chickens and a few other farm animals. They were very poor and mostly lived off the land, except for the occasional livestock that they would sell in town. I remember her telling me a story of when her brother was sick, and they had to bring him to the town hospital. He needed surgery and the family had to sell their biggest cow to pay for it. He needed medicine after the surgery and her family would go into the town every month to the church's free clinic to pick up the medicine. Sometimes, the church would run out of it and he would have to go a few months without medicine until they could get more.

As I listened to Rosa's stories, I felt like I wanted to go back in time and help her and her family, somehow. I knew that wasn't possible, but I already knew that I wanted to go into healthcare. So I decided that I would try my best to get involved and do global health work. It has been my dream to travel to Central America and help people like Rosa. I hope that I will be able to participate on next semester's global health rotation.

Michael's global health rotation essay

Thank you for considering my application to participate in next semester's global health rotation. I have never participated on a global health trip before but I feel like I would be a great fit for this rotation. Even though my career will take place in an advanced US healthcare system, I feel like I will learn a lot from an experience practicing medicine in a resource poor environment. I feel very strongly about the medical NGO's mission to not only provide immediate care for underserved communities by setting up temporary clinics, but also help them develop longstanding infrastructure. I look forward to participating in their water filtration projects in addition to the time spent in clinic. My experience in the Boy Scouts taught me a lot about wilderness survival, the importance of only drinking clean water, and different techniques for purifying water. In PA school we have learned about how diarrhea from unclean drinking water is one of the top killers of children in the world. So a clean water infrastructure that will remain after we leave is definitely as important as temporary clinics.

I am a strong team player and I think that I will fit in well with the group. I traveled a lot with my high school football team and I was always the one trying to keep the guys positive. I understand that travelling in big groups can be very challenging and the conditions in rural Central America are difficult. I am always happy to contribute and willing to do a number of different jobs in order to help things run smoothly.

Professor Rosen looked over at Sarah and started munching on his half of the muffin.

"So what do you think?" he asked.

"Wow," she said, readjusting the glasses on her nose, "they're very different."

"They certainly are," he said, "so, why don't we start with your initial impressions?"

"Well, Kelsey has a great story," she said, "her essay is well written and flows very nicely. I really liked it when I read it. But then I read Michael's essay, and he didn't have an interesting story to tell, and it wasn't even written that well. But something about it made me feel like, he had a better handle on this."

"Ah," he said, while raising one finger in the air, "so let's dig into that more. What do you think gave you that feeling?"

Sarah took off her glasses and folded them into her lap. She looked up at the ceiling and stared for a few moments. Professor Rosen patiently sipped his cappuccino.

"For one, Michael was able to talk about specific things he would do on the medical trip," Sarah started, "like he understands what he was getting into. He didn't just say he wanted to go and help people, like Kelsey did. Michael talked about the temporary clinics and he specifically named the water filtration project as something he was particularly interested in."

"I agree," he said, "what else?"

"I like how he was able to tie everything in with some personal experience," she continued, "like how he had worked with water filters before in the Boy Scouts. His remark about travelling with the high school football team was a little corny, but at least it made me feel like I was getting to know him. Boy Scouts, Football, I am starting to build an image of what Michael is like and what he is about."

"Very good," he said, "I totally agree with you. We get a sense of his personality that we just don't get from Kelsey's essay. And were you able to pick up anything from their essays about motivations and intentions?"

"Kelsey certainly said she was motivated. Her personal story with Rosa was great. I felt for Rosa's family and that little boy, but I am not sure she understood the scope of what she was getting into. Michael's point about diarrhea being one of the top killers of children in the world really hit home. It made me want to cheer him on and say, 'Yes! You go put in those water filters!' As far as intentions, Kelsey didn't mention anything about what she would do while she was there. But Michael really sounded like he wanted to fully participate in all aspects of the trip and be productive. Even though he had never been on a trip before, he was already trying to think about what he could bring to the experience and contribute to the team, not just what he would get out of it, personally."

"So if you had to pick your team members for a medical trip," Professor Rosen asked, "and I gave you these two essays without ever having met the students, would you pick Kelsey or Michael to go with you?"

"That is such a difficult decision," Sarah said, putting her hand on her chin. "Kelsey might very well be a brilliant student who would totally outperform Michael on any clinical rotation, but I just don't feel like I know anything about her from her essay. She just didn't give me enough to judge her on. Michael, on the other hand, seems well informed, motivated, excited, friendly, and driven. And having been a Boy Scout he could probably start a fire if we ever needed one!" she laughed.

"I really hope you are getting the point of what I've tried to show you, here," Professor Rosen said, "altruism, self-fulfillment, and gaining medical knowledge were great themes that we *expected* to see in these essays. What would set them apart was the personal piece that each student could bring to it. Some students did a better job than others at displaying their motivations, intentions, and understanding of the global health rotation.

Professor Rosen took the last bite of his muffin and washed it down with a sip of his cappuccino.

"You know," he continued, "a majority of the personal statements that applicants write for admission to a variety of programs in the health professions fall into one or several of the following categories:

- A dramatic story about delivering care
- A story of personal illness or caring for a loved one with an illness
- The desire to provide care for others
- Fascination with science and medicine
- Stories about working in the healthcare system

And I want to point out that just because many essays talk about similar themes doesn't mean they are inevitably trite. For example, it makes perfect sense that many people applying to a health profession would choose to talk about a desire to care for others. What isn't helpful to an admissions committee is when the applicant simply states, "I always knew, ever since I was very young, that I wanted to care for people" because it doesn't really tell us anything about the applicant. It would be more helpful for that person to describe their experiences caring for people and the context they were in. Anything that helps the reader pick up on the applicant's personality, motivation, and fit. Then, the applicant's desire to care for people would be implicit within the essay. That is what the essay is all about. It is not a writing competition, it is a personal pitch."

"Like a business pitch?" she asked.

"Exactly," he said. "When you are writing an essay like this, or a personal statement, or a cover letter for a job application, you are selling yourself. You are trying to convince the reader that you are the best person for the job."

"Oh, I'm not good at bragging," Sarah interrupted.

"And you shouldn't brag," he snapped back, "there is nothing worse than an arrogant applicant. But bragging and showcasing your strengths are two different things. If the reader thinks that you want someone to hand you a PA license right away because you are *already* overqualified, then you are bragging, and your application will wind up in the trash. But if you showcase your unique qualities, tell the reader some key things about yourself, and explain why you are motivated to do this, you will shine."

Professor Rosen paused for a moment to gather his thoughts. He continued, "You have to keep in mind, as you already noticed, each

PA application can easily be dozens of pages in length and wonderful pieces of information can be lost on the reader as they sift through hundreds of applications. For example, if you speak a second language or you won a special award or you are an author on a manuscript, or you struggled through an educationally underserved background and overcame difficult life challenges, it needs to come out in your essay, even though you have already checked the appropriate box and listed them in their designated spaces. You should not be afraid of selling yourself boldly by pitching your accomplishments and positive attributes. The essay is not the place to be shy and if you are careful you can do this without being pompous. So, for example, if you were to say that you are a highly experienced lab researcher, you would sound arrogant. But if you were to say that the work you did in a lab gave you the chance to coauthor a manuscript that was published, you would sound impressive."

"OK, so basically," Sarah started while clasping her hands together, "after reading my essay, you feel like you don't really know anything about me. I haven't talked about my background or my experience. I talked a little bit about why I want to become a PA but it was pretty vague and generic. I didn't showcase any special strengths or unique talents. I just tell this great story about one of my patients but I don't really talk about who I am and what I'm about."

"You're getting it!" he said with a smile. "The bottom line is this: your personal statement tells the story *of* you, not just a story *about* you."

"Got it," Sarah said while grabbing her bag, "thank you so much again for meeting with me. I am going back to the drawing board."

THE FINAL DRAFT

"GOOD JOB, SARAH," PROFESSOR ROSEN SAID IN the last of their meetings, "I really think that your personal statement has come a long way. You do a good job of pitching yourself by showcasing your unique talents and accomplishments. Your personality comes through, your motivations are clear, and your experience is appropriate. I think this would be a great essay to put in your application. Good luck!"

Sarah's essay. Final Draft

New England is my home. I grew up just outside of Boston in a sleepy suburban town and went to college not too far away. Every fall, as the foliage burned bright shades of orange, yellow, and red, I would hunker down with my textbooks and start the new academic year with vigor after returning to campus from my summer camp job. I spent most of the years since junior high school as a summer camp counselor but the last few years, I spent in the camp's clinic. I received my EMT certification during the end of my freshman year. I had been waiting impatiently to turn eighteen so that I could finally join the ranks of the camp's medical staff. I was drawn to that role for as long as I can remember. It felt gratifying to take care of the cut, scraped, burned, overheated campers, and anything else that would walk through the doors. I already knew that I wanted to be a PA, so I read and learned as much as

I could while I was there and tried to pitch in as much as possible. I was very honored to have received a leadership award at the end of my last year for my efforts in reorganizing the clinic's health records system.

I am very close with my family and going away to college was a difficult transition. My first year in school didn't go exactly as planned. There was an adjustment period to campus life and I was frequently travelling home to visit with my grandmother. She had lived with us for several years and she has Parkinson's disease. I learned a good bit about neurology just by going to various medical visits with her. It was hard to get away from her and the rest of my family, but when she saw that my grades were suffering, she told me, "Sarah, you can't just waste away your dream of becoming a primary care provider by spending all your time at home. You have to invest in yourself in order to give back."

So I took her advice to heart. I really invested myself in my coursework towards the end of my first year. I focused on my goal and I was able to make the Dean's list every semester since then.

My last year in college, I became a nurse's aide and started working at a rehabilitation facility. It was very different from the sprains and insect bites I had been seeing at summer camp. Many of these patients reminded me of my grandmother and I would often find myself, at the end of a shift, sitting at the piano in the recreation room and playing some music to try to brighten the atmosphere and regale them a little.

I shadowed several different health professionals as part of my pre-health circuit to gain a better understanding of their roles but I always knew that I wanted to be a PA. The PAs I shadowed always had the most well rounded understanding of the health system, the patient, and the plan. Pat is a PA who works in a primary care medical home model. When I was shadowing Pat, even when we would see a complex patient along with the physician, she would always stay in the room, after the physician left, to answer questions and help coordinate care. Everyone in the medical home clinic: doctors, nurses, pharmacists, front office staff; they would all come to Pat when they needed something. Pat was like the glue that held the clinic together.

Pat became a role model and a mentor to me. I tried to apply some of the lessons I learned to my rehab facility job and began developing broader relationships with the nurses, therapists, and other nursing assistants. It started by just learning their names and saying hello. Eventually, I gained a better understanding of their roles and their workflows. I was able to figure out that if I timed some of the patients' bed baths and vitals at just the right intervals, I was able to get everyone to and from their therapy sessions so that no one was late. The nurse manager noticed my efforts and I was honored with a Patient Care Excellence Award a few months ago.

I enjoy working on healthcare teams. I love the medical home model because of its collaborative and interprofessional philosophy. If given the opportunity to attend PA school, I would like to help develop a collaborative and friendly learning environment among my fellow students. I look forward to a career as a primary care PA and I would also like to work in a medical home model, like Pat. Thank you for considering my application.

REFERENCES

Alvarez S. Arguing academic merit: meritocracy and the rhetoric of the personal statement. *Journal of Basic Writing*. 2012:32–56.

Benkins LK, Huckin TN, Kijak L. The Personal Statement in Medical School Applications: Rhetorical Structure in a Diverse and Unstable Context. *Issues in Writing*. 2004;15(1):56–75.

Brown G, Imel B, Nelson A, Hale LS, Jansen N. Correlations between PANCE performance, physician assistant program grade point average, and selection criteria. *The Journal of Physician Assistant Education*. 2013;24(1):42–44.

Crane JT, Ferraro CM. Selection Criteria for Emergency Medicine Residency Applicants. *Academic Emergency Medicine*. 2000;7(1):54-60.

Ding H. Genre analysis of personal statements: Analysis of moves in application essays to medical and dental schools. *English for Specific Purposes*. 2007;26(3):368-392.

Dong T, Kay A, Artino AR, et al. Application Essays and Future Performance in Medical School: Are They Related? *Teaching and Learning in Medicine*. 2013;25(1):55-58.

Ferguson E, McManus IC, James D, O'Hehir F, Sanders A. Pilot study of the roles of personality, references, and personal statements in relation to performance over the five years of a medical degree Commentary: How to derive causes from correlations in educational studies. *BMJ*. 2003;326(7386):429–432.

Forister JG, Jones PE, Liang M. Thematic analysis of personal statements in physician assistant program admissions. *The Journal of Physician Assistant Education*. 2011;22(2):6–12.

GlenMaye L, Oakes M. Assessing suitability of MSW applicants through objective scoring of personal statements. *Journal of Social Work Education*. 2002;38(1):67–82.

Higgins R, Moser S, Dereczyk A, et al. Admission variables as predictors of PANCE scores in physician assistant programs: a comparison study across universities. *The Journal of Physician Assistant Education*. 2010;21(1):10–17.

Jones PE, Simpkins S, Hocking JA. Imperfect physician assistant and physical therapist admissions process in United States of America. *Journal of Educational Evaluation for Health Professions*. 2014;11:11.

Kirchner GL, Stone RG, Holm MB. Use of Admission Criteria to Predict Performance of Students in an Entry-Level Master's Program on Fieldwork Placements and in Academic Courses. *Occupational Therapy In Health Care*. 2001;13(1):1-10.

Lee AG, Golnik KC, Oetting TA, et al. Re-engineering the Resident Applicant Selection Process in Ophthalmology: A Literature Review and Recommendations for Improvement. *Survey of Ophthalmology*. 2008;53(2):164-176.

Lopes JE, Badur M, Weis N. How Physician Assistant Programs Use the CASPA Personal Statement in Their Admissions Process: *The Journal of Physician Assistant Education*. 2016;27(2):51-55.

Lopes Jr JE, Delellis NO, DeGroat A, Jacob N. An analysis of theme content in CASPA personal statements. *The Journal of Physician Assistant Education*. 2014;25(4):43–46.

Mathur A, Kamat D. The Personal Statement. *The Journal of Pediatrics*. 2014;164(4):682-682.e1.

Max BA, Gelfand B, Brooks MR, Beckerly R, Segal S. Have personal statements become impersonal? An evaluation of personal statements in anesthesiology residency applications. *Journal of Clinical Anesthesia*. 2010;22(5):346-351.

McDaniel MJ, Hildebrandt CA, Russell GB. Central Application Service for Physician Assistants Ten-Year Data Report, 2002 to 2011. *The Journal of Physician Assistant Education*. 2016;27(1):17–23.

O'Neill LD, Korsholm L, Wallstedt B, Eika B, Hartvigsen J. Generalisability of a composite student selection programme. *Medical Education*. 2009;43(1):58-65.

Peskun C, Detsky A, Shandling M. Effectiveness of medical school admissions criteria in predicting residency ranking four years later. *Medical Education*. 2007;41(1):57-64.

Sadler J. Effectiveness of student admission essays in identifying attrition. *Nurse Education Today*. 2003;23(8):620-627.

Shulruf B, Wang YG, Zhao YJ, Baker H. Rethinking the admission criteria to nursing school. *Nurse Education Today*. 2011;31(8):727-732.

Smith EA, Weyhing B, Mody Y, Smith WL. A Critical Analysis of Personal Statements Submitted by Radiology Residency Applicants1. *Academic Radiology*. 2005;12(8):1024-1028.

Thrasher A. Factoring leadership into the admissions process. *The Journal of Physician Assistant Education*. 2012;23(2):49.

Warner ML, Maio C, Hudmon KS. Career patterns of physician assistants: A retrospective longitudinal study. *Journal of the American Academy of Physician Assistants*. 2013;26(6):44-48.

ABOUT THE AUTHOR

Dr. Berkowitz is the Director of Research and a founding faculty member of the Boston University School of Medicine Physician Assistant Program. He holds a PhD in Epidemiology from the University of Pittsburgh and has practiced for many years as a PA in neurosurgery. Dr. Berkowitz is a researcher and a medical educator who has published numerous works in healthcare research journals as well as a medical fiction novel. He lives with his wife and son in Boston, Massachusetts.

Also by Oren Berkowitz
The Brain Surgeon, a medical fiction novel

www.DrOrenBerkowitz.com

94499657R00037

Made in the USA
Lexington, KY
30 July 2018